Decoding the Enigma of Memory

Navigating the Landscape of Alzheimer's Disease

Shirley L. Brooks

Table of contents

Introduction

 Welcome to the fascinating realm of cognition and memory. In this exploratory excursion, we dig into the complexities of quite possibly the most baffling issue that influences the human psyche - Alzheimer's sickness.

Alzheimer's infection, a moderate and crushing neurodegenerative condition, has spellbound the consideration of researchers, clinical experts, and guardians all over the planet. A complicated riddle difficulties how we might interpret memory and its significant effect on our very quintessence as people.

We will provide a brief overview of Alzheimer's disease in this introduction, laying the groundwork for a more in-depth investigation of its enigmatic landscape. An excursion intends to uncover the secret mysteries and shed light on the colossal difficulties faced by those impacted by this neurological issue.

Picture a scene where loved recollections, once energetic and striking, start to disappear. A person's ability to remember precious moments, recognize loved ones, and navigate the world they once knew so well is eroded as a result of Alzheimer's disease, which steals bits and pieces of their identity.

The scientific foundations that define Alzheimer's disease will be examined as we delve deeper into the disease. We will investigate the multifaceted systems that drive the beginning and movement of the infection, unwinding the intricacies that encompass it.

However, this journey is not just about the scientific and clinical aspects. It is likewise a journey into the close-to-home and individual components of Alzheimer's sickness. As individuals, families, and communities navigate the difficulties of supporting and caring for Alzheimer's patients, we will witness the profound impact on them.

Through the course of this investigation, we will experience accounts of versatility, compassion, and trust. We will observe the victory of the human soul as guardians and specialists work enthusiastically to open the privileged insights of this illness, endeavoring to work on the existences of those impacted and eventually track down a fix.

Thus, go along with us as we leave on this edifying and sympathetic excursion - Opening the Secrets of Memory: Exploring the Scene of Alzheimer's Infection. Step into a domain where science and mankind meet, acquiring a more profound comprehension of this complicated problem and the steady assurance to vanquish it.

Alzheimer's illness is a perplexing and moving scene to explore. Millions of people worldwide are affected by this progressive neurological disorder, which results in memory loss, cognitive decline, and behavioral changes. As we dive into this scene, it is vital to move toward it with sympathy, understanding, and a guarantee to track down arrangements.

One of the critical parts of exploring the scene of Alzheimer's illness is instruction. People and those close to them can better deal with the challenges posed by the disease if they are aware of its symptoms and progression. In addition, gaining knowledge of the most recent research and treatment options can offer hope and direction for managing the disease.

Support is one more critical component in exploring this scene. Parental figures, relatives, and companions assume an essential part in giving close-to-home, physical, and down-to-earth help to those residing with Alzheimer's. People with the disease may benefit from guidance, resources, and a sense of community through professional services, online communities, and support groups.

Notwithstanding instruction and backing, imagination and versatility are fundamental while exploring the scene of Alzheimer's. Tracking down imaginative ways of imparting, drawing in, and animating people with Alzheimer's can extraordinarily upgrade their satisfaction. Some creative methods that can help Alzheimer's patients connect with their memories and emotions include music therapy, art therapy, and memory activities.

In addition, technology plays a significant role in navigating the Alzheimer's disease landscape. From wearable gadgets that track day-to-day exercises and screen well-being to brilliant home frameworks that advance security and freedom, innovation offers a scope of answers to help people with Alzheimer's and their parental figures.

Finally, to navigate the Alzheimer's disease landscape, it is essential to advocate for increased awareness, funding, and research. By raising public mindfulness, we can diminish shame and advance comprehension. Expanded subsidizing can uphold research endeavors pointed toward tracking down a fix or growing more powerful medicines. Backing can likewise prompt approach changes that further develop admittance to focus and back on those impacted by Alzheimer's.

Even though navigating the Alzheimer's disease landscape can be difficult, it is essential to keep in mind that there is hope. Through schooling, support, imagination, innovation, and backing, we can affect the existence of those impacted by this staggering sickness.

We can work together to improve care, find a cure, and eventually eradicate Alzheimer's disease from the world.

Significance and impact on individuals and society

Step into a world where our memories create the intricate tapestry of our lives and serve as the foundation of our identities. Now, picture that tapestry slowly falling apart, one thread at a time. This is the significant effect of Alzheimer's sickness on people and society in general.

Alzheimer's sickness, a tireless neurological issue, has arisen as one of the main difficulties within recent memory. Its compass reaches out a long way past the individual impacted, saturating families, networks, and social orders in general. Its effect swells through the texture of our social design, requesting consideration and understanding.

We examine the significance and far-reaching effects of Alzheimer's disease in this introduction, highlighting its profound effects on individuals and society. We open a door into a world in which memories slip through our fingers like grains of sand as we investigate its emotional, financial, and social implications.

Alzheimer's sickness strikes at the actual center of our human experience. Our self-perception is distorted as a result of its symptoms, which gradually erase precious memories, leaving a void that cannot be filled. The friends and family wrestling with this sickness get through a lamentable excursion as they witness the disintegration of their valued connections and the departure that could only be described as epic of shared encounters.

However, the effect is even more extensive. As the pervasiveness of Alzheimer's infection rises, social orders are confronted with critical financial and care loads. Families navigate the emotional toll of being a caregiver, healthcare options, and the intricate maze of financial decisions. Policymakers face the challenge of providing sufficient support and resources while the burden of caring for an aging population strains health systems.

However, there is hope amidst this impact on society. People impacted by Alzheimer's illness, their families, specialists, and guardians have met up in a chorale of versatility and assurance. They look for ways to stop, slow down, and eventually cure this relentless disease as they try to unravel the mysteries of memory.

We want to shed light on the significance of Alzheimer's disease and the profound effects it has on individuals and society through this investigation. We will explore the close-to-home scene, giving sympathy and understanding to those contacted by this infection. We will investigate the financial outcomes and the critical requirement for coordinated endeavors to help those impacted and track down a way forward.

As we investigate the mysteries of memory, navigate the terrain of Alzheimer's disease, and work toward a future in which memories can flourish unaffected by this devastating disorder, we invite you to join us on this illuminating journey. Let us strive, collectively, for a world free of Alzheimer's disease, where memories are treasured and the true essence of who we are can endure.

The importance and effect of Alzheimer's illness on people and society couldn't possibly be more significant. At a singular level, Alzheimer's can be obliterating, denying people their recollections, freedom, and capacity to perform day-to-day undertakings. It can create turmoil, dissatisfaction, and a feeling of misfortune for both the people living with the infection and their friends and family.

The effect on society is likewise significant. Healthcare systems, caregivers, and the economy as a whole suffer greatly from Alzheimer's disease. The expense of really focusing on people with Alzheimer's is faltering, with gauges arriving at billions of dollars every year. This incorporates clinical costs, long-haul care, and lost efficiency because guardians find employment elsewhere or decrease their functioning hours to give care.

In addition, people with Alzheimer's disease are impacted not only by themselves but also by their loved ones and friends. As they navigate the challenges of providing care, caregivers frequently experience high levels of stress, burnout, and financial strain. The profound cost of seeing a friend or family member decay can be colossal, prompting sensations of pain, responsibility, and disengagement.

Due to an aging population, it is anticipated that the prevalence of Alzheimer's disease will significantly rise in the coming years on a societal level. This will overwhelm medical care frameworks, social administrations, and assets. It features the pressing requirement for expanded mindfulness, exploration, and backing to address the developing effect of Alzheimer's on society.

Nonetheless, it is essential to take note that amid the difficulties, there is likewise versatility, strength, and trust. People living with Alzheimer's can in any case track down snapshots of bliss, association, and reason. Comfort, understanding, and a sense of community can be provided by caregivers and support networks. Society can unite to push for change, support research, and enhance the lives of Alzheimer's patients.

By perceiving the importance and effect of Alzheimer's illness, we can pursue a future where people get the consideration and support they merit, where exploration prompts leap forwards in treatment and counteraction, and where society is better prepared to explore the scene of Alzheimer's with sympathy, empathy, and understanding.

Chapter 1: Understanding Alzheimer's

Welcome to the world of understanding Alzheimer's, where we embark on a journey into the intricate workings of the human brain and the profound mysteries of memory.

At the heart of Alzheimer's disease lies a complex interplay between the brain's structure, function, and the fragile threads of memory. In this exploration, we aim to unravel the basics of brain function and memory, laying a foundation for comprehending the enigma that is Alzheimer's.

The human brain, with its billions of interconnected neurons, acts as the command center of our bodies and the keeper of our memories. It is a marvel of nature, orchestrating our every thought, action, and emotion. Within this intricate organ, synapses fire, neurotransmitters transmit signals, and memories are formed and stored.

Memory, one of the brain's most extraordinary abilities, allows us to recall past experiences, learn from our mistakes, and shape our sense of self. It encompasses various forms, from the immediate recollection of an event to the retention of information over time. It is the fragile yet resilient tapestry that weaves the fabric of our lives.

To understand Alzheimer's disease, we must first comprehend the intricacies of memory. Memories are created through a complex process involving multiple regions of the brain working in harmony. The hippocampus, an essential structure nestled deep within the brain, plays a central role in the formation and consolidation of memories.

However, in Alzheimer's disease, this delicate balance is disrupted. The hallmark characteristics of the disease, the accumulation of abnormal proteins called beta-amyloid plaques and tau tangles, wreak havoc on the brain. These disruptions interfere with the communication between neurons, deteriorating synaptic connections and impairing memory function.

As Alzheimer's disease progresses, individuals may experience a range of memory-related symptoms. Mild forgetfulness, difficulty with word recall, and challenges in problem-solving may be early signs of cognitive decline. Over time, as the disease advances, memory loss becomes more pronounced, causing individuals to struggle with familiar tasks, recognize loved ones, and even maintain basic self-care abilities.

However, understanding Alzheimer's disease goes beyond knowing the symptoms. It requires delving deeper into the complexities of brain function and memory. Researchers strive to unlock the mechanisms underlying this disease, seeking to develop treatments that can halt or slow its progression.

In this exploration of Alzheimer's disease, we will journey into the fascinating world of the brain and memory, discovering the vital processes that shape our cognitive abilities. We will unravel the key functions of different brain regions, such as the hippocampus and cerebral cortex that are profoundly affected by Alzheimer's disease.

Together, let us delve into the nuances of brain function and memory, expanding our understanding of the basic foundations disrupted by Alzheimer's disease. Through knowledge and empathy, we aim to foster support, advance research, and ultimately work towards a future where this devastating disease is conquered and memories can once again flourish.

How Alzheimer's affects the brain

The progressive brain disorder known as Alzheimer's disease affects millions of people worldwide. It is the most considered normal reason for dementia, a term used to depict a decrease in mental capacities sufficiently extreme to obstruct day-to-day existence. To develop effective treatments and offer assistance to individuals with Alzheimer's disease and their families, it is essential to comprehend how the disease affects the brain.

Through intricate networks, billions of nerve cells, or neurons, in a healthy brain communicate with one another. These neurons have specific designs called neurotransmitters, which permit them to communicate electrical and compound signs. They cooperate to handle data, structure recollections and have different mental capabilities.

Notwithstanding, in Alzheimer's illness, these fundamental associations between neurons are disturbed and in the long run, obliterated. The sickness essentially influences two kinds of unusual designs in the mind: amyloid plaques and tau tangles.

Beta-amyloid protein clumps that form outside neurons are known as amyloid plaques. These proteins are normally broken down and disposed of, but in Alzheimer's disease, they build up and form sticky plaques. These plaques make it hard for neurons to communicate with one another, making it harder for them to effectively send signals.

In contrast, tau tangles are twisted tau protein fibers that accumulate within neurons. Tau proteins are fundamental for keeping up with the construction of neurons and working with the vehicle of supplements and other fundamental substances. However, in Alzheimer's disease, these proteins become abnormal and clump together, leading to cell death and the breakdown of the neuron's transport system.

As the illness advances, the harm brought about by amyloid plaques and tau tangles spreads all through the cerebrum, especially in regions critical for memory, learning, and thinking. The hippocampus, a locale liable for framing new recollections, is much of the time one of the principal regions impacted. This makes sense of why cognitive decline and disarray are early side effects of Alzheimer's.

As the illness progresses, different locales of the cerebrum, for example, the cerebral cortex, which controls language, thinking, and social way of behaving, additionally become impacted. Changes in behavior and personality are a result of this, as are difficulties in communication and problem-solving.

Moreover, the mind's general size and construction likewise change in Alzheimer's illness. The cortex, which is liable for higher mental capabilities, contracts, and the ventricles, which are liquid-occupied spaces, grow. This deficiency of cerebrum tissue adds to the ever-evolving decrease in mental capacities found in Alzheimer's patients.

While the specific reason for Alzheimer's illness is as yet not completely perceived, research recommends a blend of innate, biological, and lifestyle factors to add to its new development. Age is the main gambling factor, with most cases happening in people more than

65 years of age. However, people in their 40s and 50s can also develop early-onset Alzheimer's.

Understanding how Alzheimer's influences the cerebrum is vital for creating successful medicines and medications. To halt or stymie the disease's progression, researchers are actively testing a variety of strategies, such as targeting tau tangles and amyloid plaques. In addition, managing the difficulties associated with the disease requires assisting and caring for people with Alzheimer's and their families.

In conclusion, Alzheimer's disease is a complicated neurological condition that changes how the brain looks and works. The gathering of amyloid plaques and tau tangles disturbs correspondence between neurons, prompting mental degradation and cognitive decline. We can work toward developing better Alzheimer's treatments and support systems for those affected by the disease by expanding our knowledge of it.

Causes and risk factors

The reasons for Alzheimer's sickness are not yet completely comprehended, yet specialists have distinguished a few factors that might assume a part in its turn of events.

1. **Age:** The most significant risk factor for Alzheimer's disease is getting older. The majority of people who develop Alzheimer's disease are 65 or older, and the risk doubles every five years after 65.

2. **Genetics:** The risk of Alzheimer's disease has been linked to particular genes. Individuals with a family background of the condition are bound to foster it themselves. The most notable quality is called Apolipoprotein E (APOE), with variations of APOE4 expanding the gamble.

3. **The family tree:** Having a parent or kin with Alzheimer's infection builds a singular gamble of fostering the condition.

4. **Way of life and cardiovascular variables:** Undesirable way of life decisions like smoking, absence of actual activity, less than stellar eating routine, and corpulence might expand the gamble of Alzheimer's illness. Furthermore, conditions that influence cardiovascular well-being, similar to hypertension, elevated cholesterol, and diabetes, may add to the improvement of Alzheimer's

5. **Head injury:** Supporting huge head wounds, especially rehashed blackouts, has been

connected to a higher gamble of fostering Alzheimer's sickness sometime down the road.

6. **Constant illnesses:** Certain constant circumstances, including coronary illness, stroke, and misery, have been related to an expanded gamble of Alzheimer's.

7. **Ecological elements:** Although more research is needed to fully comprehend these potential links, environmental toxins like pesticides or heavy metals may contribute to Alzheimer's disease development.

It is essential to take note that while these variables increment the gamble, they don't ensure that a singular will foster Alzheimer's infection.

Chapter 2: Early Detection and Diagnosis

Alzheimer's infection is an ever-evolving cerebrum problem that slowly influences memory, thinking, and conduct. There are numerous reasons why early Alzheimer's diagnosis and detection are so important. It makes it possible for people and their families to get the right medical care, make plans for the future, and use support services. Perceiving the early signs and side effects is vital to distinguishing the sickness in its underlying stages.

Cognitive decline is one of the most well-known and conspicuous side effects of Alzheimer's infection. However, it is essential to keep in mind that forgetfulness on occasion is a typical symptom of aging. In the beginning phases of Alzheimer's, people might encounter trouble recollecting late scholarly data, significant dates, or occasions. They might also forget conversations they had just minutes ago, rely heavily on memory aids or repeatedly ask for the same information.

One more early indication of Alzheimer's is trouble with critical thinking and arranging. People might find it trying to follow a recipe, deal with their funds, or complete errands that require different advances. They might battle with focus, take more time to finish natural responsibilities or commit more errors than expected.

Additionally, language difficulties may be a sign of early Alzheimer's disease. People might experience difficulty tracking down the right words to put themselves out there or battle-to-follow discussions. Additionally, they might have trouble reading, writing, or comprehending written information.

Changes in temperament and character can likewise be early admonition indications of Alzheimer's sickness. People might become bad-tempered, restless, or discouraged for reasons unknown. Additionally, they may exhibit behavioral changes, such as withdrawing from previously enjoyable social activities or becoming more easily agitated.

Notwithstanding these mental and conduct changes, people may likewise encounter actual side effects in the beginning phases of Alzheimer's. They might experience issues with coordination, experience balance issues, or experience difficulty with spatial mindfulness. They may likewise show changes in their rest designs, like sleep deprivation or unnecessary daytime drowsiness.

Perceiving these early signs and side effects of Alzheimer's illness can be a challenge, as they can be unpretentious and handily credited to typical maturing or different variables. Nonetheless, it is critical to focus on diligent or demolishing side effects and look for clinical guidance assuming there are concerns.

Clinical experts utilize various appraisals and tests to analyze Alzheimer's infection. A comprehensive medical history, a physical examination, cognitive tests, and brain imaging scans are all examples of these. For a precise diagnosis, it's critical to talk to a doctor who specializes in memory disorders.

Early location and determination of Alzheimer's illness offer a few advantages. It enables individuals and their families to access support services, make well-informed choices regarding medical care and treatment options, and plan for the future. It likewise gives a potential chance to take part in clinical preliminaries and examination studies pointed toward tracking down better medicines and eventually a solution for Alzheimer's.

In conclusion, early diagnosis and detection of Alzheimer's disease need to recognize its early symptoms. Physical symptoms, mood and personality changes, memory loss, and difficulty solving problems can all be signs of the disease. Looking for clinical guidance and counseling an expert in memory problems is fundamental for an exact finding and to get to proper consideration and backing administrations. Early detection contributes to ongoing Alzheimer's disease research and gives individuals and their families the ability to make educated decisions and plans for the future.

Importance of timely diagnosis

The opportune determination of Alzheimer's infection is of most extreme significance for people and their families. Distinguishing the sickness in its beginning phases considers better administration of side effects, admittance to proper clinical consideration, and the valuable chance to anticipate what's in store. Understanding the significance of convenient analysis can essentially influence the existence of those impacted by Alzheimer's.

One of the essential advantages of early recognition is the capacity to get to clinical consideration and treatment choices that can assist with dealing with the side effects of Alzheimer's. Although there is no cure for the disease at this time, early intervention can halt its progression and enhance quality of life. Some treatments and medications can temporarily improve symptoms, cognitive function, and day-to-day functioning.

People and their families can make plans for the future when they get a diagnosis early. Alzheimer's is a disease that gets worse over time and progresses. By being familiar with the conclusion right off the bat, people can come to significant conclusions about their consideration inclinations, legitimate and monetary issues, and long-haul care choices. This eases the burden on family members who may be required to make decisions on their behalf and allows them to influence their destiny.

Besides, the convenient conclusion empowers people and their families to get help administrations and assets custom-made for Alzheimer's patients. Support gatherings, advising administrations, and instructive projects can offer close-to-home help and viable guidance for adapting to the difficulties related to the illness. Respite care and assistance with managing the day-to-day care needs of loved ones can also be beneficial to caregivers.

Early finding likewise permits people to partake in clinical preliminaries and exploration studies. Scientists are continually making progress toward tracking down better medicines and at last a solution for Alzheimer's. By taking part in clinical preliminaries, people add to progressing logical information and have the chance to get to trial medicines that may dial back or stop the movement of the sickness.

Besides, convenient determination diminishes nervousness and vulnerability for the two people and their families. It gives a reason for the changes in behavior and cognitive function that might have been worrying. It permits people to more readily comprehend their condition, look for suitable help, and foster survival techniques to deal with the difficulties they might confront.

Last but not least, early Alzheimer's disease detection and diagnosis raise awareness among healthcare providers, policymakers, and the general public. It features the significance of examination, subsidizing, and assets committed to Alzheimer's consideration and backing. Additionally, it aids in the reduction of stigma and fosters empathy and comprehension for those living with the disease.

Taking everything into account, the significance of the ideal conclusion of Alzheimer's illness couldn't possibly be more significant. It makes it possible to get medical care, treatments, and support services that can make life better. It enables individuals and their families to make informed decisions and plan for the future. A timely diagnosis also aids in Alzheimer's disease research and raises public awareness. By perceiving the meaning of early recognition, we can all the more likely help and care for those impacted by this staggering condition.

Disease progression

Alzheimer's infection is an ever-evolving neurological turmoil that influences the mind, especially the regions liable for memory, thinking, and conduct. This degenerative condition progressively deteriorates after some time, prompting huge mental degradation and useful disabilities. We should investigate the overall movement of Alzheimer's infection for quite a while.

Early stage (Mild Cognitive Impairment):

In the beginning phases, people might encounter unobtrusive changes in memory and mental capacities. Mild Cognitive Impairment (MCI) is a common name for this stage. Forgetfulness, difficulty solving problems, and occasional confusion are some of the more typical symptoms. Some people may not be aware of these symptoms, but standardized memory tests typically reveal them. During this stage, people can in any case play out their day-to-day exercises autonomously, yet they might find specific errands seriously testing.

Middle stage (Mild to Moderate Alzheimer's):

As Alzheimer's illness advances to the center stage, the side effects become more observable and start to affect everyday working all the more fundamentally. As memory loss gets worse, people may forget their names and faces, get lost in familiar places, and have trouble communicating. They might encounter trouble with direction, show changes in character and conduct, and display issues with rest designs. During this stage, people frequently need more help and management with their day-to-day exercises, including individual consideration and well-being.

Late stage (Moderate to severe Alzheimer's):

In the late phase of Alzheimer's, very serious mental degradation happens, making it provoking for people to perceive friends and family and convey actuality. People may be unable to recall recent events or even their personal history when memory loss becomes severe. They might need consistent help with individual considerations, like washing, dressing, and eating. Conduct changes are normal, including tumult, meandering, dreary developments or discourse, and expanded trouble with coordinated movements. In this stage, people are exceptionally subject to guardians for all parts of everyday living.

End stage (Severe Alzheimer's): Alzheimer's disease:

In the last phase of Alzheimer's, people frequently lose the capacity to answer their current circumstances, articulate their thoughts, or control their development. They might end up in bed and have trouble swallowing, making them more likely to get sick. Because the individual is completely dependent on others for all activities of daily living during this stage, it is necessary to provide care round-the-clock. It's critical to take note that the term of each stage can fluctuate and the movement of Alzheimer's sickness can contrast from one individual to another.

While there is as of now no solution for Alzheimer's illness, medicines can assist with overseeing side effects, dial back the movement, and work on personal satisfaction for certain people. Support from medical services suppliers, parental figures, and care groups can be pivotal in giving help, direction, and basic reassurance for both the individual and their friends and family through the different phases of this difficult illness.

Chapter 3: Current Treatment Approaches

Current Treatment Approaches for Alzheimer's: Medications and Therapies

While there is no cure for Alzheimer's disease, several treatment approaches are available to help manage symptoms, slow down the progression of the disease, and improve the quality of life for individuals living with Alzheimer's. These approaches primarily include medications and various therapies that target different aspects of the disease.

Medications play a crucial role in the treatment of Alzheimer's disease. They can temporarily alleviate symptoms, improve cognitive function, and enhance daily functioning. The most commonly prescribed medications for Alzheimer's are cholinesterase inhibitors and memantine.

Cholinesterase inhibitors, such as donepezil, rivastigmine, and galantamine, work by increasing the levels of acetylcholine, a chemical messenger involved in memory and learning, in the brain. These medications help improve cognitive function, including memory, thinking, and reasoning. They can also alleviate some behavioral and psychological symptoms of Alzheimer's.

Memantine, on the other hand, works by regulating the activity of another chemical messenger called glutamate. It helps improve cognitive function, especially in the later stages of Alzheimer's, and may also help manage behavioral symptoms.

In addition to medications, various therapies are available to support individuals with Alzheimer's and their families. These therapies aim to improve cognitive function, enhance communication, manage behavioral symptoms, and promote overall well-being. A portion of the normally utilized treatments include:

1. **Cognitive Stimulation Therapy (CST):** CST involves engaging individuals in group activities and discussions that stimulate memory, attention, and problem-solving skills. It aims to improve cognitive function and enhance social interaction.

2. **Reality Orientation Therapy (ROT):** ROT uses visual aids, calendars, and other cues to help individuals with Alzheimer's maintain a sense of time, place, and personal identity. It can reduce confusion and improve orientation.

3. **Reminiscence Therapy:** This therapy involves discussing past experiences, looking at old photographs, and engaging in activities that evoke memories. Reminiscence therapy can improve mood, enhance communication, and provide a sense of identity and self-worth.

4. **Music and Art Therapy:** Music and art therapy can have a positive impact on individuals with Alzheimer's. Listening to familiar music or engaging in art activities can reduce agitation, improve mood, and stimulate memories and creativity.

5. **Behavioral Therapies:** Behavioral therapies focus on managing behavioral symptoms, such as agitation, aggression, and wandering. These therapies involve identifying triggers, modifying the environment, and using techniques like redirection and validation to address challenging behaviors.

It is important to note that treatment approaches may vary depending on the stage and severity of Alzheimer's disease and the individual's specific needs. Healthcare professionals, including neurologists, geriatricians, and psychiatrists, play a crucial role in assessing symptoms, prescribing appropriate medications, and recommending therapies tailored to each individual.

While current treatments for Alzheimer's focus on managing symptoms and improving quality of life, ongoing research is exploring new approaches and potential breakthroughs. Scientists are investigating novel medications, immunotherapies, and lifestyle interventions that may slow down or even prevent the progression of the disease.

In conclusion, current treatment approaches for Alzheimer's disease primarily involve medications and various therapies. Medications, such as cholinesterase inhibitors and memantine, aim to improve cognitive function and manage symptoms. Therapies, including cognitive stimulation, reality orientation, reminiscence, and music/art therapy, focus on enhancing cognitive abilities, communication, and overall well-being. While these treatments cannot cure Alzheimer's, they play a crucial role in managing symptoms and improving the quality of life for individuals living with the disease. Ongoing research continues to explore new treatment options and potential breakthroughs in the fight against Alzheimer's.

Lifestyle modifications for management

Current Treatment Approaches for Alzheimer's: Way of Life Adjustments for the Board

Notwithstanding meds and treatments, way of life changes assume a huge part in the administration of Alzheimer's sickness. The purpose of these alterations is to enhance cognitive function, enhance overall health, and enhance the quality of life for people with Alzheimer's disease. Integrating sound propensities and making specific way of life changes can emphatically affect dealing with the side effects of the sickness.

1. **Customary Actual Activity:** Taking part in standard actual activity has been displayed to have various advantages for people with Alzheimer's. Exercise boosts cognitive function, increases new neuron formation, and increases blood flow to the brain. Additionally, it may lower the risk of cardiovascular diseases and other Alzheimer's-related health conditions.

2. **Healthy eating:** An even and nutritious eating routine is fundamental for cerebrum wellbeing. Healthy fats, whole grains, lean proteins, and fruits and vegetables are all good sources of the nutrients your brain needs to function properly. A few examinations propose that the Mediterranean eating regimen, which stresses plant-based food varieties, fish, and solid fats, may decidedly affect mental capability and lessen the gamble of Alzheimer's.

3. **Mental Excitement:** Keeping the mind dynamic and connected through mental feeling can assist with keeping up with mental capability. Exercises like perusing, puzzles, acquiring new abilities, and taking part in friendly connections can animate the mind and possibly delay mental deterioration. It is essential to open doors to mental excitement and participate in exercises that challenge the cerebrum consistently.

4. **Quality Rest:** Sleeping enough and getting enough of it is important for your mental and physical health. Unfortunately, rest can add to memory issues and deteriorate mental side effects in people with Alzheimer's. Laying out a normal rest schedule, establishing an agreeable rest climate, and rehearsing great rest cleanliness can advance better rest quality.

5. **Stress The board:** Cognitive function and general well-being can be negatively affected by chronic stress. Tracking down viable pressure the executive's methods, for example, unwinding works out, profound breathing, contemplation, and participating in pleasant exercises, can assist with diminishing feelings of anxiety and work on close-to-home prosperity.

6. **Social Connection:** Keeping up with social associations and taking part in significant social exercises can emphatically affect people with Alzheimer's. Social cooperation invigorates the cerebrum, further develops the state of mind, and lessens sensations of seclusion and sadness. One's overall well-being needs to encourage participation in social activities, join support groups, and build relationships with friends and family.

7. **Security Measures:** Executing security estimates inside the living climate is urgent for people with Alzheimer's. This might incorporate eliminating possible dangers, guaranteeing appropriate lighting, utilizing assistive gadgets, and executing methodologies to forestall meandering and falls.

It is critical to take note that way of life changes ought to be carried out related to clinical medicines and treatments endorsed by medical services experts. The needs and abilities of each person with Alzheimer's disease should be taken into consideration when developing a treatment plan.

Changes in one's lifestyle can't stop Alzheimer's, but they can help manage symptoms better, improve one's well-being as a whole, and even slow down cognitive decline. Embracing a solid way of life and rolling out sure improvements can engage people with

Alzheimer's and their families to effectively partake in their consideration and boost their satisfaction.

In conclusion, changes to one's lifestyle are an important part of the current Alzheimer's disease treatment. Customary actual activity, a solid eating regimen, mental feeling, quality rest, stress the executives, social commitment, and security estimates all add to the administration of side effects and general prosperity. By consolidating these way of life adjustments, people with Alzheimer's can upgrade their mental capability, keep up with their freedom, and work on their general personal satisfaction.

Managing Alzheimer's disease

Dealing with Alzheimer's infection includes a thorough methodology that spotlights on dialing back the movement of side effects, working on personal satisfaction, and offering help for the two people with Alzheimer's and their guardians. The following are some important aspects of managing Alzheimer's disease:

1. **Medication:** Drugs supported by administrative offices, like cholinesterase inhibitors (donepezil, rivastigmine, galantamine) and memantine, can assist with overseeing side effects and dial-back mental degradation. These drugs work by expanding synapses in the

cerebrum, further developing memory and thinking skills. When choosing the best medication and dosage, it is essential to consult a medical professional.

2. **Cognitive Stimulation:** Reading, solving puzzles, and engaging in hobbies are all examples of mind-expanding activities that can assist in extending cognitive abilities. Mental feelings, including memory games and social communication, may work on general mental capability and personal satisfaction. Mental recovery programs, frequently driven by word-related specialists, can likewise be valuable.

3. **Physical Exercise:** Standard active work has been found to have various advantages for people with Alzheimer's sickness. Exercise can work on by and large actual well-being, upgrade state of mind, and advance better rest. It might likewise assist with lessening mental degradation by expanding the bloodstream to the cerebrum and invigorating the development of new synapses. Before beginning an exercise program, it is essential to consult a medical professional.

4. **Nutritional Management:** An even eating routine that incorporates organic products, vegetables, entire grains, lean proteins, and

sound fats is fundamental for generally speaking well-being and cerebrum capability. Additionally, a lower risk of cognitive decline has been linked to certain dietary patterns like the Mediterranean diet, which includes foods high in omega-3 fatty acids and antioxidants. For individualized dietary recommendations, it is essential to consult a registered dietitian or other medical professional.

5. **Caregiver Support:** Caregivers of Alzheimer's patients can face significant stress due to the disease, so it is essential to provide them with sufficient assistance. This can incorporate rest care, guidance, and schooling about the sickness and its movement. Support bunches explicitly for guardians can offer important everyday reassurance, pragmatic tips, and an organization of people encountering comparable difficulties.

6. **Safety Precautions:** Safety measures become increasingly important as Alzheimer's disease progresses. This may entail implementing fall prevention strategies, reducing wandering behaviors by securing the home environment, and ensuring that Alzheimer's patients do not run the risk of ingesting harmful substances by accident. Using advances like wearable GPS

trackers and home observing frameworks can likewise upgrade security.

7. **Social and emotional support:** Emotional and social isolation can be significant effects of Alzheimer's disease. Empowering proceeds with a commitment to friendly exercises, keeping up with connections, and offering close-to-home help can enormously work on prosperity. Mental and social mediations, like memory treatment and music treatment, can likewise assist with animating positive feelings and further developing a state of mind.

For Alzheimer's illness, the executives require a complex methodology that consolidates clinical administration, solid way of life decisions, parental figure backing, and social commitment. Normal coordinated effort with medical services experts, including nervous system specialists, geriatricians, and partnered wellbeing suppliers, is significant in creating customized care designs and changing therapy procedures on a case-by-case basis.

Caregiving Challenges

Caregiving Alzheimer's patients presents a particular set of difficulties. It can be a rewarding and important job, but it also takes a lot of physical, emotional, and mental energy. Caretakers frequently encounter the following problems:

1. **Progressive Nature of the Illness:** Alzheimer's is an ever-evolving illness, implying that the side effects and care needs of a singular will strengthen over the long haul. Caregivers often find themselves under more and more pressure as the disease progresses, necessitating constant adjustments to their methods and approaches to providing care.

2. **Mental and Conduct Changes:** Alzheimer's can cause tremendous changes in comprehension and conduct, making correspondence, and understanding testing. Parental figures might experience challenges in attempting to speak with people with Alzheimer's, as they might experience difficulty putting themselves out there or perceiving their friends and family. Changes in behavior, like agitation, aggression, and depression, can also be a big problem for caregivers.

3. **Physical Demand:** As the sickness advances, people with Alzheimer's might need help with exercises of everyday living, including washing, dressing, toileting, and eating. This puts an actual weight on guardians, as they frequently

need to furnish involved care and help with versatility.

4. **Emotional Stress:** Being a caregiver for an Alzheimer's patient can be emotionally draining. Seeing a friend or family member decay, encountering trouble and pain over their cognitive decline, and overseeing testing ways of behaving can prompt parental figure burnout, nervousness, and misery. The loss of previous relationship dynamics and the sensation of being constantly "on call" can exacerbate the emotional toll.

5. **Financial Burden:** The expenses related to giving consideration to a person with Alzheimer's can be significant. Clinical costs, home changes to guarantee well-being and expert consideration administrations can strain a guardian's funds. Adjusting the monetary obligations close to providing care can cause extra pressure and uneasiness.

6. **Isolation and Social Impact:** Providing care can now and again prompt disengagement, as parental figures might have restricted investment in their public activities and individual undertakings. The consistent requests to provide care can make it challenging to keep

up with connections or take part in exercises that bring individual satisfaction. Caregiver exhaustion and feelings of loneliness can be exacerbated by social isolation.

7. **Lack of Support:** Numerous parental figures might feel overpowered and unsupported as they explore the intricacies of Alzheimer's consideration. The absence of mindfulness and understanding from others, restricted admittance to assets and administrations, and lacking relief care choices can additionally strain guardians.

Parental figures should look for help, both viable and close to home, to adapt to these difficulties. This might include connecting with help gatherings, looking for rest care, getting too instructive assets, and using accessible local area administrations. Parental figures ought to likewise focus on taking care of themselves, like enjoying reprieves, looking for relief, keeping up with their well-being, and looking for help from loved ones. Finding solutions to Alzheimer's caregiving problems and managing them can be made easier with open communication with healthcare professionals and a strong support network.

Impact of Alzheimer's Disease on Mental Health

Memory, thinking, and behavior are all affected by the progressive neurological disorder known as Alzheimer's disease. It not only essentially affects mental capability but also influences emotional wellness in different ways. Here are a portion of the effects of Alzheimer's sickness on emotional well-being:

1. **Depression:** Sorrow is a typical psychological wellness issue experienced by people with Alzheimer's infection. The deficiency of memory, autonomy, and capacity to perform day-to-day exercises can prompt sensations of bitterness, sadness, and uselessness.

2. **Anxiety:** Nervousness problems, for example, summed up tension confusion, and social uneasiness issues, can create because of Alzheimer's sickness. The vulnerability about the future, challenges in correspondence, and the feeling of dread toward failing to remember significant data or individuals can add to expanded tension levels.

3. **Disturbance and animosity:** Alzheimer's infection can cause social changes, including expanded unsettling and hostility. These alterations can be distressing for both the Alzheimer's patient and those who care for them, resulting in increased stress and challenges with mental health.

4. **Isolation from others and loneliness:** As Alzheimer's sickness advances, people might pull out from social exercises and connections because of troubles in correspondence and cognitive decline. This can hurt mental health by making people feel lonely and socially isolated.

5. **Problems falling asleep:** Sleep patterns are frequently disrupted by Alzheimer's disease, resulting in insomnia or excessive daytime sleepiness. Mental well-being can be negatively impacted by poor-quality sleep, which can increase irritability, confusion, and mood swings.

6. **Loss of personality and confidence:** Alzheimer's infection can make people lose their self-appreciation and way of life as their recollections and capacities decline. This

misfortune can bring about low confidence, sensations of disarray, and a reduced feeling of direction, influencing emotional wellness.

7. **Parental figure trouble:** The effect of Alzheimer's infection on emotional wellness isn't restricted to the people with the condition; it additionally influences their parental figures. Focusing on somebody with Alzheimer's infection can be genuinely and sincerely requested, prompting expanded pressure, tension, and misery among guardians.

It is vital to address the psychological wellness effects of Alzheimer's infection through fitting mediations and emotionally supportive networks. This might include directing, support gatherings, medicine, and way-of-life adjustments to work on general prosperity for the two people with Alzheimer's and their guardians.

Chapter 4: Ongoing Research and Breakthroughs

Alzheimer's infection is a staggering neurodegenerative problem that influences a great many individuals around the world. Nonetheless, there is progressing research and various leap forwards that give the desire to better grasp, determination, and treatment of this condition. As of late, researchers and clinical experts have gained huge headway in disentangling the secrets encompassing Alzheimer's, prompting promising turns of events.

The discovery of potential biomarkers for early detection is one of the most exciting discoveries in Alzheimer's research. Early determination is critical for successful mediation and treatment, as it considers the execution of treatments that can dial back or stop the movement of the illness. Specialists have found that particular proteins, like amyloid-beta and tau, play a huge part in the improvement of Alzheimer's. Doctors can identify individuals at risk of developing the disease before symptoms appear by detecting these proteins in the cerebrospinal fluid or using imaging techniques.

One more area of promising improvement is the investigation of novel remedial methodologies. Customary medication medicines for Alzheimer's have shown restricted achievement, yet late investigations have uncovered possible leaps forward. For example, scientists are researching the utilization of monoclonal antibodies to target and eliminate amyloid-beta plaques, which are accepted to be a sign of Alzheimer's. These antibodies have shown promising outcomes in early clinical preliminaries, offering expected powerful sickness-changing therapies later on.

Besides, progressions in innovation and man-made consciousness have opened up new roads for Alzheimer's examination. AI calculations are being created to examine enormous datasets, including hereditary data, cerebrum imaging, and clinical information, to recognize examples and potential gambling factors for Alzheimer's. This approach can upset how we might interpret the illness and help in the improvement of customized treatment plans.

Notwithstanding these forward leaps, scientists are likewise investigating non-pharmacological intercessions to work on the personal satisfaction of people with Alzheimer's. Mental preparation programs, actual activity, and social commitment have been shown to guarantee to dial back mental deterioration and working on general prosperity.

Overall, Alzheimer's disease research is producing promising results that give hope for improved diagnosis, treatment, and management. We can strive for a time when Alzheimer's is no longer a debilitating disease but instead, a condition that can be effectively managed and treated with continued dedication and collaboration among scientists, medical professionals, and caregivers.

Potential future treatments and interventions

Alzheimer's disease affects millions of people worldwide and is a complicated and devastating condition. Our efforts to develop potential future treatments and interventions are advancing at the same rate as our understanding of the disease.

One likely road for future medicines is the investigation of novel medication treatments. Targeting specific proteins involved in the development of Alzheimer's disease, such as amyloid beta and tau, is one strategy being investigated by researchers. It is hoped that disease progression can be slowed or even stopped by developing drugs that effectively reduce the accumulation of these proteins or prevent their harmful effects.

One more encouraging area of examination is the utilization of immunotherapies. These medicines intend to bridle the force of the insusceptible framework to perceive and clear unusual proteins related with

Alzheimer's. By animating a resistant reaction against these proteins, scientists accept it could be feasible to dial back or even converse the mental deterioration found in Alzheimer's patients.

Moreover, headways in quality treatment hold a guarantee for future mediations. Researchers are looking into ways to fix or replace defective genes that cause Alzheimer's disease. It may be possible to delay or prevent the disease's onset by focusing on specific genes.

Also, there is a developing interest in non-pharmacological medications for Alzheimer's illness. These include alterations to one's way of life, physical activity, and cognitive training. Research recommends that participating in intellectually animating exercises, keeping a sound eating routine, and guaranteeing standard actual work can decidedly affect mental capability and possibly decrease the gamble of fostering Alzheimer's.

It is essential to keep in mind that further research and clinical trials are required to validate the safety and efficacy of these potential future treatments and interventions, even though they offer hope. The excursion towards finding viable medicines for Alzheimer's illness is progressing, and the coordinated effort between researchers, medical care experts, and backing bunches stays critical in our mission to work on the existence of those impacted by this staggering condition.

Benefits of targeting specific proteins in the development of Alzheimer's disease

Focusing on unambiguous proteins in the improvement of Alzheimer's illness can offer a few possible advantages. Beta-amyloid is one of the main proteins linked to Alzheimer's disease. It forms plaques in the brain by targeting specific proteins. Researchers hope to achieve several benefits by targeting this protein in the development of Alzheimer's disease. Beta-amyloid plaques, which may assist in slow load, which forms plaques, in slowing the progression of Alzheimer's disease, are one of the key proteins that prevent or remove these plaques associated with the disease.

One more protein of interest is tau, which in the cerebrum is accepted to add to structures tangles in the mind the movement of the illness. By focusing on. Focusing on tau could beta-amyloid, analysts at any point forestall the development of this knot and safeguard the desire to forestall or lessen the arrangement of these synapses from harm. Plaques, have the potential to either slow down or even stop the progression of the disease.

Another protein-induced disease development.

Other proteins that are involved in Alzheimer's disease include tau, which makes tangles like ApoE4 and causes inflammation in the brain, both of which are features of related proteins. Focusing on being read up for their likely job in the tau could assist with forestalling the arrangement of this t improvement and movement of the sickness. Target angles and the subsequent damage caused by these proteins to brain cells may contribute to their cause.

By focusing on unambiguous lessening aggravation and advancing mind wellbeing.

In general, researchers hope to halt or slow down Alzheimer's disease by focusing on specific proteins involved in the disease. They also hope to identify the underlying processes that lead to the development of treatments that can alter the underlying disease, which causes brain cell degeneration and cognitive process, and to improve cognitive function decline in Alzheimer's disease. This approach has memory, and generally personal satisfaction for people with Alzheimer's. The possibility to give indicative help as well as possibly adjust the course it's critical to take note of that further exploration is expected to completely comprehend the sickness, working on by and large results for people the job of these proteins and foster protected and powerful treatments impacted by Alzheimer's. Notwithstanding, it's essential to take note that further exploration and clinical preliminaries are expected to completely comprehend the viability and well-being of focusing on these proteins.

Chapter 5: Coping Strategies for Patients and Caregivers

Survival techniques for patients and parental figures of Alzheimer's illness are fundamental for dealing with the difficulties and stresses that accompany this dynamic neurological issue. Alzheimer's infection presents deterrents for both the people analyzed and their friends and family who take on providing care obligations.

It is essential to develop coping mechanisms for Alzheimer's patients that emphasize preserving independence and enhancing cognitive function. Daily life experiences can be enhanced by having structured routines and a supportive environment. The following are a couple of survival methods for patients:

1. **Participate in mental excitement:** Reading, puzzles, and memory games can all help maintain cognitive abilities and improve brain health.

2. **Keep yourself healthy:** Normal activity, a reasonable eating regimen, and adequate rest add to general prosperity, which can decidedly influence mental capability.

3. **Influence memory helps:** Utilizing schedules, updating applications, and electronic coordinators can assist with mitigating memory-related difficulties.

4. **Stress management techniques:** Exercises like profound breathing activities, reflection, and unwinding procedures can diminish nervousness and further develop adapting capacities.

5. **Look for social connection:** Taking part in bunch exercises, support gatherings, or get-togethers can battle separation and proposition consistent reassurance.

For guardians of people with Alzheimer's infection, it is urgent to focus on taking care of oneself and layout survival techniques that diminish pressure and forestall burnout. Caregivers can use these coping mechanisms:

1. **Instruct yourself:** Finding out about the illness and understanding its movement can provide guardians with information and better prepare them to give proper consideration.

2. **Create a support system:** Joining a parental figure support bunch or interfacing with different guardians

can offer close-to-home help, useful counsel, and a feeling of the local area.

3. **Be realistic about your goals:** Accept that you cannot accomplish everything on your own. Caregiver burnout can be avoided by allowing others to assist and delegating tasks.

4. **Enjoy standard reprieves:** Plan time for taking care of oneself and participate in exercises that bring unwinding and restoration.

5. **Obtain services for respite care:** Utilize respite care programs, whether provided by professional caregivers or trusted friends and family. These administrations permit guardians to have a break while their cherished one gets suitable consideration.

6. **Counseling or therapy can help you deal with stress:** Looking for proficient assistance can give you a place of refuge to communicate feelings, learn new methods for dealing with hardship or stress, and foster successful correspondence strategies.

7. **Acceptance training and celebrating small victories:** Recognize that the infection advances over the long run and that the patient's capacities might decline. Concentrate on savoring everyday moments and recognizing small victories.

The goal of these coping mechanisms is to improve the quality of life for Alzheimer's patients and those who care for them. It is essential to recall that every individual's involvement in this sickness is novel and acclimations to ways of dealing with hardship or stress might be important as the condition advances. Looking for help and direction from medical services experts can help with fitting survival methods to address explicit necessities and difficulties.

Support systems and resources

Emotionally supportive networks and assets assume an imperative part in helping people with Alzheimer's illness and their guardians deal with the difficulties related to the condition. Throughout the journey, these support systems offer information, emotional support, practical assistance, and direction. Here are some key emotionally supportive networks and assets accessible for Alzheimer's infection:

1. **Alzheimer's Affiliations:** Associations like the Alzheimer's Relationship (in the US) and Alzheimer's General Public (in the Unified Realm) give an abundance of assets and backing administrations. These affiliations offer helplines, instructive materials, support gatherings, and online networks that associate people and guardians confronting comparative difficulties.

2. **Professionals in the medical field and memory clinics:** Memory centers represent considerable authority in diagnosing and overseeing memory issues, including Alzheimer's sickness. These centers offer complete evaluations, treatment choices, and direction for the two patients and guardians.

3. **Support gatherings:** People with Alzheimer's disease and those who care for them can find a safe and supportive environment in which to share their experiences, get advice, and learn coping skills by joining local or online support groups.

4. **Programs for respite care:** Rest care administrations offer transitory alleviation to guardians by giving proficient help and backing to their friends and family. These projects can give present moment providing care alleviation either at home or in proficient consideration offices, permitting guardians to enjoy reprieves and take care of their necessities.

5. **Grown-up day care focuses:** During the day, these centers provide Alzheimer's patients with a secure and stimulating setting. They offer organized programs, social collaboration, and regulated exercises to advance mental capability and give reprieve to parental figures.

6. **Services for home care:** In the comfort of the patient's own home, trained caregivers can assist with

daily activities, personal care, medication management, and companionship.

7. **Monetary and lawful assets:** Assistance with insurance, benefits, long-term care planning, and legal documentation such as powers of attorney and advance healthcare directives are among the many resources available to assist families in navigating the financial and legal aspects of Alzheimer's disease.

8. **Prescription and treatment assets:** The most recent information on medications, clinical trials, and treatment options for managing Alzheimer's disease symptoms can be accessed through consultations with healthcare professionals, such as neurologists and geriatric specialists.

9. **Assistive advancements and security measures:** To help people with Alzheimer's disease and the people who care for them, a variety of technological tools and safety precautions have been developed. These can incorporate GPS beacons, medicine-the-board applications, home-checking frameworks, and versatile gear to upgrade freedom and security.

10. **Instructive assets:** Information about Alzheimer's disease, its stages, caregiving strategies, and resources are the subject of numerous books, online forums, websites, and educational programs. These assets

enable people and parental figures with information and better prepare them to give proper consideration.

It is essential to keep in mind that support systems and resources may vary from country to country. To find the most up-to-date and relevant support services, individuals and caregivers should look into local resources specific to their location and consult with healthcare professionals.

Enhancing quality of life for those affected

Increasing the quality of life for those with Alzheimer's disease should be a top priority in coping strategies for patients and caregivers. Despite the challenges posed by the disease, these strategies aim to boost well-being, preserve independence, and cultivate meaningful connections. Here are a few survival methods that emphasize upgrading personal satisfaction for people with Alzheimer's sickness and their parental figures:

1. **Concentrate on the remaining skills:** Patients and caregivers alike can concentrate on the Alzheimer's patient's remaining abilities and strengths. By distinguishing and taking part in exercises that use these capacities, a feeling of direction and achievement can be kept up. For instance, assuming the individual appreciates painting, they might participate in more

worked-on workmanship exercises that take special care of their abilities to ongoing.

2. **Participate in significant exercises:** Empowering people with Alzheimer's to participate in exercises they appreciate can improve their satisfaction. These exercises could incorporate paying attention to music, planting, partaking in delicate activities, or playing prepackaged games. Maintaining cognitive function and emotional well-being can be aided by engaging in enjoyable and familiar activities.

3. **Create a routine for your day:** For people with Alzheimer's, establishing and sticking to a daily routine can provide a sense of structure and stability that can be comforting. This includes keeping a steady timetable for feasts, cleanliness schedules, proactive tasks, and relaxation exercises. An established routine can lessen anxiety and confusion.

4. **Establish a supportive atmosphere:** Changing the actual climate can add to improving the personal satisfaction of people with Alzheimer's. Using visual navigational aids like labeled drawers or color-coded objects, reducing clutter, ensuring good lighting, and minimizing noise are all important aspects of creating a supportive and safe environment.

5. **Encourage social associations:** Keeping up with social associations can extraordinarily improve the

prosperity of people with Alzheimer's. Energize visits from loved ones, take part in get-togethers or care groups, and focus on friendly cooperation as a component of the singular's everyday practice. Social commitment can offer profound help, lessen disconnection, and animate mental capability.

6. **Practice viable correspondence:** Adapting communication strategies can be beneficial for both patients and caregivers. Understanding can be improved and frustration reduced by employing clear, simple language, and visual cues, and maintaining nonverbal communication (such as touch or facial expressions). Effective communication necessitates patient listening and active listening.

7. **Focus on taking care of oneself for guardians:** Guardians should focus on taking care of oneself to upgrade their prosperity. This could mean looking into respite care, taking frequent breaks, participating in activities they enjoy, and seeking assistance from friends, family, or support groups. Keeping up with their own physical and close-to-home well-being is fundamental for furnishing quality consideration to the person with Alzheimer's.

8. **Be educated and seek information:** The two patients and guardians benefit from instructing themselves about Alzheimer's infection. Grasping the sickness' movement, side effects, and accessible help

and assets can assist people and parental figures with feeling more engaged and better prepared to oversee difficulties.

9. **Put stress-management strategies into practice:** Stress management is important for both patients and caregivers. Taking part in pressure decrease exercises like reflection, profound breathing activities, yoga, or participating in leisure activities can assist with lessening tension and advance unwinding.

10. **Look for proficient direction:** Experts in the field of Alzheimer's disease medicine, such as doctors, therapists, and social workers, can offer helpful advice and resources. They can provide individualized strategies to address specific challenges and improve quality of life.

Every individual's involvement in Alzheimer's illness is novel, and methodologies might be adjusted as the sickness advances. As a result, improving the quality of life for Alzheimer's patients and those who care for them requires a tailored, adaptable strategy.

Chapter 6: Raising Awareness and Advocacy

1. **Dissipating confusions:** There are a lot of misconceptions about Alzheimer's disease, such as the idea that it is just memory loss or that it is a normal part of getting older. By educating the general public about the disease's complex nature and its effects on cognitive function, behavior, and day-to-day functioning, raising awareness helps dispel these misconceptions.

2. **Advancing early location and determination:** Further developed public comprehension can urge people to look for clinical consideration assuming they notice concerning memory or mental changes. Interventions, treatments, and support services that can improve quality of life and possibly halt the progression of the disease are made possible by early detection.

3. **Empowering compassion and backing:** Public comprehension encourages sympathy and empathy for people living with Alzheimer's and their guardians. It assists individuals with perceiving the difficulties they face and urges the local area to offer help,

understanding, and incorporation for those impacted by the infection.

4. **Promoting funding and research:** Expanded mindfulness can help make a groundswell of public help for Alzheimer's examination. Support endeavors can provoke policymakers and financing associations to focus on research subsidizing, prompting leap forwards in figuring out the sickness, further developing therapy choices, and endeavoring towards tracking down a fix.

5. **Decreasing shame and seclusion:** In reducing the stigma associated with Alzheimer's disease, public understanding is crucial. People with Alzheimer's and their caregivers are less likely to be judged and to feel alone when accurate information is shared, creating a supportive environment that encourages them to be active members of society.

6. **Upgrading backing and assets:** A very educated public is bound to search out and use accessible emotionally supportive networks and assets for Alzheimer's illness. Expanded mindfulness can prompt the turn of events and extension of encouraging groups of people, instructive projects, and administrations that take special care of the interesting necessities of people with Alzheimer's and their guardians.

7. **Enabling parental figures:** Policies that help caregivers can be implemented sooner if people are made aware of the difficulties they face. This incorporates admittance to reprieve care administrations, monetary help, work environment facilities, and parental figure-preparing programs. A more proficient public can advocate for better help and assets to reduce the weight put on guardians.

8. **Collaboration with healthcare professionals:** Better communication between healthcare providers and the general public is made possible by public awareness. By engaging people and guardians with information about Alzheimer's sickness, they become dynamic members in their medical services venture, adding to additional educated choices and further developed results.

9. **Creating public talk:** An educated society takes part in conversations about Alzheimer's illness, and its effect on people, families, and networks. Public mindfulness can animate discussions about the requirement for arrangements, expanded research, further developed dementia-accommodating conditions, and comprehensive networks, at last, driving cultural change.

10. **Connecting with media and celebrities:** Joining forces with news sources and VIPs who have individual encounters with Alzheimer's can be a strong

method for bringing issues to light and a promoter for a bigger scope. They can use their platforms to help spread messages to a wider audience and motivate people to take action.

Bringing issues to light and backing for Alzheimer's infection is a continuous exertion that requires joint efforts between people, associations, medical services experts, scientists, policymakers, and the media. We can build a society that understands, empowers, and supports people with Alzheimer's and their caregivers by educating the public, dispelling myths, and encouraging empathy and support.

Advocacy efforts for increased research and support

Dedicated efforts to promote increased funding for Alzheimer's research and assistance for those affected by the disease are necessary for raising awareness and advocating for the condition. Support assumes a vital part in driving strategy changes, impacting regulation, and preparing assets to work on the existences of those living with Alzheimer's and their guardians. The following are important points highlighting the advocacy efforts for increased Alzheimer's disease research and support:

1. **Advancing examination subsidizing:** Backing endeavors center around bringing issues to light of the

significance of Alzheimer's exploration and pushing for expanded subsidizing from government organizations, confidential establishments, and partnerships. Expanded research subsidizing considers noteworthy disclosures, progressions in treatment choices, and at last, draws us nearer to tracking down a fix.

2. **Interacting with decision-makers:** Promotion includes drawing in policymakers at neighborhood, public, and worldwide levels to guarantee Alzheimer's sickness stays a need on their plans. Advocates can gain support for increased funding, improved healthcare policies, and enhanced caregiver support programs by educating policymakers about the disease's impact on individuals and society.

3. **Collaboration with academic institutions:** Advocacy groups support the efforts of research institutions and organizations to investigate Alzheimer's disease. To accelerate progress in understanding the disease, they advocate for the allocation of resources, streamlining research procedures, and fostering collaboration among various institutions and fields.

4. **Increasing awareness:** Backing endeavors expect to raise public mindfulness about the effect of Alzheimer's illness, its commonness, and the pressing requirement for research subsidizing and support

administrations. Advocacy groups can foster a sense of urgency and widespread support for the Alzheimer's crisis by increasing public understanding.

5. **Supporting parental figure assets and administrations:** Advocacy includes pushing for more resources and services that are tailored to caregivers' needs. This might include upholding relief care programs, parental figure preparing drives, support gatherings, and monetary help programs that reduce the physical, close-to-home, and monetary weight looked at by guardians.

6. **Driving strategy changes:** Policy changes that benefit Alzheimer's patients and their caregivers are the goal of advocacy efforts. This might include pushing for approaches that further develop admittance to medical care administrations, advance early finding and mediation, safeguard the freedoms and pride of people with Alzheimer's, and make steady and comprehensive networks.

7. **Working together with backing associations:** Organizations and advocacy groups collaborate to promote common objectives and increase their impact. By working together and pooling assets, promotion endeavors can contact a more extensive crowd, influence mastery, and make a durable voice in upholding expanded exploration and backing.

8. **Drawing in mainstream researchers:** To comprehend the most recent developments in Alzheimer's disease research, advocates collaborate closely with scientists, researchers, and healthcare professionals. This joint effort assists advocates with remaining informed, sharing basic data with people in general, and giving input on research needs that line up with the requirements of people impacted by Alzheimer's.

9. **Activating grassroots endeavors:** The grassroots support and participation of affected individuals, caregivers, families, and community members are essential to advocacy. Advocates can cultivate a groundswell of support that exerts pressure on policymakers and raises awareness of the requirement for research funding and support by mobilizing grassroots efforts, raising awareness at the local level, and organizing community events.

10. **Using media and innovation:** Promotion endeavors influence different correspondence channels, including conventional media, virtual entertainment, and online stages, to disperse data, share individual stories, and rally public help. Advocates can reach a large number of people, interact with key stakeholders, and have an impact that lasts a lifetime by utilizing these channels.

Promotion endeavors for expanded exploration and backing are persistently advancing and require steady and supported activity. By bringing issues to light, captivating policymakers, supporting exploration organizations, and building solid local area organizations, promoters can drive the vital changes expected to work on the existences of people living with Alzheimer's sickness and their guardians.

Conclusion

In conclusion, unlocking the mysteries of memory and navigating the landscape of Alzheimer's sickness requires a purposeful exertion from people, associations, medical care experts, policymakers, and the more extensive local area. We can appreciate the significance of this endeavor by recapitulating key points:

1. There are numerous stigmas and misconceptions regarding Alzheimer's disease. Bringing issues to light is significant in scattering these confusions and advancing exact comprehension of the illness.

2. Early identification and conclusion are urgent in dealing with Alzheimer's sickness. Expanded public comprehension can incite people to look for clinical consideration and access mediation and backing administrations that can improve their satisfaction.

3. Sympathy and backing assume a fundamental part in offering care and understanding to those living with Alzheimer's and their parental figures. Public comprehension can cultivate sympathy and inclusivity, diminishing the shame and detachment related to the infection.

4. To obtain funding for research, advocacy efforts are essential. Expanded financing empowers leap forwards in grasping the sickness, further developing therapy choices, and pursuing tracking down a fix.

5. Policy and legislation may be altered as a result of public understanding. Engaging policymakers, influencing policy modifications, and setting priorities for the resources and assistance that Alzheimer's patients require are all aided by advocacy.

6. Lessening shame and cultivating steady networks are necessary for people impacted by Alzheimer's. By sustaining an educated society, we can guarantee sufficient assets, steady organizations, and comprehensive conditions that take care of the interesting necessities of people living with Alzheimer's and their parental figures.

7. Coordinated effort is key in bringing issues to light and pushing for expanded examination and backing. By joining forces with research establishments, medical care experts, and promotion associations, and

utilizing media and innovation, we make a strong voice that impels change.

Unlocking the mysteries of memory Opening the secrets of memory and navigating the landscape of Alzheimer's sickness is a continuous excursion. We can make significant progress toward enhancing the lives of Alzheimer's patients, expediting new research findings, and fostering a society that is more compassionate and welcoming by consistently advocating for the disease and increasing public awareness. We have the power to have a long-lasting effect and give people with Alzheimer's and those who care for them hope for the future.

We must all embrace a call to action if we are to maintain the momentum in raising awareness and advancing Alzheimer's research. All of us play a part to play in having an effect. Here are a few key advances we can take to proceed with mindfulness and examination:

1. **Remain informed:** Keep up with the most recent information and developments in Alzheimer's disease research. Learn about the disease, its effects, and the state of research at the moment. Share this information with others to advance a superior grasp inside your local area.

2. **Be a champion:** Turn into a backer for Alzheimer's examination and backing. Enlist in the neighborhood or public support associations, take part in mindfulness crusades, and draw in policymakers. Support expanded financing, further developed medical services arrangements, and better help for parental figures and people living with Alzheimer's.

3. **Support research endeavors:** Add to the progressions in Alzheimer's examination by supporting associations engaged with exploration and raising assets. Donations, fundraising, and volunteering your time and skills are all options to consider. The impact of each contribution is significant.

4. **Spread mindfulness:** Spread Alzheimer's disease awareness through a variety of channels, including personal conversations, community events, and social media. Share individual stories, verifiable data, and assets to teach others and diminish the shame encompassing the illness.

5. **Draw in with medical services experts:** Keep in touch with Alzheimer's disease-specific medical professionals. Look for standard check-ups and screenings, and urge others to do likewise. Engage in proactive conversations with healthcare providers to investigate the options for support and resources that are available.

6. **Support guardians:** Provide caregivers who tirelessly care for Alzheimer's patients with support and understanding. Show appreciation for their basic job and deal with help whenever the situation allows. Learn about the resources available to caregivers and make sure they are aware of them.

7. **Encourage cooperation:** Promote collaboration among a variety of sectors, including community members, healthcare providers, policymakers, advocacy groups, and research institutions. We can bring about significant change, coordinate our efforts, and maximize our collective impact by working together.

8. **Connect with the young:** By incorporating Alzheimer's awareness and education programs into youth organizations and schools, you can educate and involve the younger generation. Empowering youthful people to become promoters and scientists will prepare for future progressions in Alzheimer's illness.

9. **Support worldwide endeavors:** Millions of people around the world are affected by Alzheimer's, which is a global problem. Ensure that international Alzheimer's organizations and initiatives receive your full support. To take a more comprehensive approach to combating the disease, collaborate with communities all over the world to share experiences, knowledge, and resources.

10. **Keep in mind your effect:** Keep in mind that every action, no matter how big or small, helps the cause. Your endeavors in bringing issues to light, supporting examination, and being a supporter can drive genuine change and affect the existences of people impacted by Alzheimer's.

By embracing this source of inspiration, we can make a strong development that keeps on bringing issues to light, advocate for expanded examination and backing, and at last pursue forestalling, treating, and restoring Alzheimer's infection. Let's work together to improve the lives of Alzheimer's patients all over the world and leave a lasting impression.